God's Prescriptions For A Healthy Society
Back to the Garden of Eden for Physical and Spiritual Renewal

GOD'S PRESCRIPTIONS FOR A HEALTHY SOCIETY
Back to the Garden of Eden for Physical and Spiritual Renewal

"What? Do you not know that your body is the temple of the Holy Spirit, Who is in you, Whom you have of God, and you are not your own? You are bought with a price! Therefore glorify God in your body, and in your spirit, which are God's" (1 Corinthians 6:19, 20 UT).

"Beloved, I pray that you may prosper in all things and be in health, just as your soul prospers" (3 John 1:2 NKJV).

by

Pastor Howard Eugene Wright

1

The gemstone for this book is an emerald.

An emerald is a rare and very valuable gemstone. In top quality varieties, fine emeralds are more valuable than diamonds. Our health is to be greatly prized. Without it we are greatly handicapped. Thus, the emerald is a fitting gemstone to represent a life that is healthy in body, soul and spirit.

God's Prescriptions For A Healthy Society

Back to the Garden of Eden for Physical and Spiritual Renewal

ISBN-10: 1479397385
ISBN-13: 978-1479397389

DEDICATION

This book is dedicated to all those of all ages who want to live an abundant life with good health in Christ Jesus, our wonderful Lord and Saviour.

ACKNOWLEDGEMENTS

I thank my wife, Arlene Roller Wright, for the hours she has spent proofreading this book and for getting the *Arlene's Kitchen* recipes ready for this book. I also thank those who have helped us find this way of spiritual and physical renewal.

PRECAUTIONS

This approach to ultimate health should NOT be done without taking heed to these precautions! It would be advisable that you have an all-body cleanse as a first step on your journey to ultimate health. This is especially true when it comes to changing your diet from processed and cooked foods to organic raw foods! Do it in stages! Carefully remove the old processed and cooked foods from your diet as you replace them with the new organic raw foods over time as your body is able to adjust to it. First, take processed and artificial sugars off and put raw honey and/or dates on. Take all cooked carbohydrates off. Then add raw carbohydrate foods. Wait a while. Then, take meats off and add nuts and seeds. You may need Vitamin B12. This can be gotten through nutritional yeast. Sea weeds, like kelp, will help you with your mineral requirements. Use natural salts. Sea salt is a good choice. These salts have minerals with them. Your physical exercise program should be done without over-stressing yourself! Start out slow and do more as you are able! Be careful not to get sunburned! Everything else in this book can be done right away with good results!

INTRODUCTION

You do have a choice! You can either have good health or bad health. You can either survive or thrive in this life. The choices you make will determine how you do both physically and spiritually. The choices you make are free for the taking. The consequences of your choices are governed by God's eternal laws. Make the wrong choices and ruin your health and fight to survive. In this sad state of affairs, you are just one breath away from death and eternity. Make the right choices and you can thrive with good health for many years to come. Then you can say with confidence, "I am not looking for the undertaker, but I am looking for the Upper-Taker, the Lord Jesus Christ, to take me to His eternal home." See John 14:1-3.

What I tell you in this book is not theory. I am a living witness, along with many others, of its value. At the age of 63, I was in very poor health. At that time, I married Arlene, a lady I had pastored 25 years earlier. My first wife died from mistakes and poor procedures used by the medical profession. Arlene's husband died the same year as my first wife. We were not planning to get married again. God had other plans. We were both trying to do a vegetarian diet with little success. Shortly after we were married we paired up with a support group that helped us do what is explained in this book. The results have been outstanding. At 74 years young, I am now in very good health. I can easily walk at a very fast pace for 10 miles without exhausting myself. The people in this little farm community are amazed at my walking ability. I do not take

6

any prescription drugs. I do not have any of the physical problems that plague other people of my age. About 2 years ago, I had two hernia surgeries. I have no scars. They have completely healed. I think better and am really enjoying life. It gets better as I go along. I feel my best years are yet ahead. Also, my relationship with God is great and getting better every day.

The problem is in the way the medical profession "treats" disease. They do one of three things: (1) drug the patient hoping to kill the "germs" before they kill the patient, (2) cut out the bad part or (3) burn it out with radiation or chemotherapy. The miracle is, some people do get well. This is a very poor way to bring people to health and well-being. Many times the side effects are worse than the disease. Furthermore, this approach hinders your body's natural healing processes.

You are indeed "fearfully and wonderfully made" as stated in Psalm 139:14. You are more than a chemical factory. God has given you a self-replicating, self-healing body. Your body is constantly replicating itself. Some cells are replaced with new ones at a faster rate than others. As a general rule, the more they are used, the faster they are replaced. Every seven (7) years your body has completely renovated itself. As you well know, the body can heal itself. We see this happening all the time. When you cut yourself it will heal over time. Furthermore, you are made up of a body, a soul and a spirit. Thus, in this book when we approach the concept of complete health we are taking into consideration the whole person.

Even though every cell in your body has the same exact genetic make-up, they are organized into specialized

7

functions. When one member suffers they all suffer. There are no "evolutionary throw-backs" in your body. Each part is necessary for it to function at its best. When any part is removed or replaced, your overall body health suffers. For example, you will die if you have no blood. Your blood must have a Ph factor of 7.4 to maintain good health. If you have too many white blood cells your health is in jeopardy. Your appendix is a very important part of your immune system. Your pituitary gland is needed to regulate many life sustaining functions in your body. Your sex organs are used for more than reproduction of the species. Every cell in your body functions with each other to maintain your health in perfect working order.

One of the basic principles to good health is to keep your immune system strong and healthy. Albert Earl Carter, in his book "*The Cancer Answer*," gives four things you need to know to keep your immune system healthy. They are: (1) cell food, (2) cell exercise, (3) cell environment, and (4) cell communication.

The pseudo-science of evolution has done you and your society great harm. Understand that true science is very limited. It has no way of answering how, when and why questions with any degree of accuracy. For example, it cannot tell you how the human race got here, when it got here and why it is here. There is only One Who can answer these question correctly. He is the One Who created all things.

Think about this. You went on a vacation. When you came home you found a UFO in your yard. The creator of the UFO is standing beside it. This being lets you know you are safe and wants to answer your how, when, and why

8

questions. What would be the best way for you to get answers to these questions? The sure way would be to ask the being standing beside the UFO. Our Creator God has done one better than this. He has given us a Book, The Holy Bible, that answers these questions. It answers them as follows: How? He spoke everything into being out of nothing. When? About 6000 years ago. Why? To bring glory and honor to Himself.

In this book I am going to address 7 prescriptions God gives us in His Word for good, high-quality life. These prescriptions' instructions are:

1. Develop a loving relationship with God.

2. Maintain a benevolent, thankful attitude toward God and others.

3. Love people in thought, word and deed.

4. Remove all resentments from your life by loving God and others.

5. Remove stress from you life by casting all your cares on God.

6. Slowly remove all processed and cooked foods from your diet.

7. Make sure all bodily and spiritual wastes are removed regularly and completely.

8. Develop a daily regular scheduled time for devotions, food, rest and exercise.

9. Eat an all-raw diet of organic vegetables, fruits, seeds, nuts, spices and herbs.

10. Daily drink one ounce of pure distilled water per two pounds of body weight.

11. Get at least eight hours of rest a day. Some need more and some less.

12. Rest with a good conscience at the end of the day.

13. Exercise on a Rebounder or have a walking program.

14. Exercise your faith and obedience toward God.

15. Get some sunlight once or twice a day.

16. Breathe fresh air as much as possible.

17. Work for your family and for the good of others.

May the Lord bless you as you learn how to take care of your wonderfully made body as well as your soul and spirit.

UT means updated text. It is changed to the modern English.

PRESCRIPTION 1 - MEANINGFUL RELATIONSHIPS

Develop a loving relationship with God. First things first! The starting point is to repent of your sins and accept the Lord Jesus Christ as your personal Savior. Sin is rebellion against God. Romans 5-12 show how you can be made a new creation in Christ Jesus. Read Matthew 5-7 to see how to live close to your Creator-Redeemer God.

"Enter in at the strait gate: for wide is the gate, and broad is the way, that leads to destruction, and many there be which go in thereat: because strait is the gate, and narrow is the way, which leads unto life, and few there be that find it" (Matthew 7:13, 14 UT).

"Do not be unequally yoked together with unbelievers. For what fellowship has righteousness with lawlessness? And what communion has light with darkness? And what accord has Christ with Belial? Or what part has a believer with an unbeliever? And what agreement has the temple of God with idols? (2 Corinthians 6:14-16b NKJV) Read 2 Corinthians 5-7:1 for a greater understanding of what is involved in walking with God.

Study your Bible, pray, witness for God, thank God for all things, learn to trust God for all your needs, obey God in every area of your life and join a Bible believing church. These are things you need to do to develop a loving relationship with your Creator-Redeemer God.

"Blessed is the man (means everyone) who has not walked in the counsel of the ungodly, and has not stood in the way of sinners, and has not sat in the seat of scorner.

11

But his delight is only in the law of the LORD, and he meditates in His law day and night" (Psalm 1:1, 2 UT).

"But you shall receive power, after that the Holy Spirit is come upon you: and you shall be witnesses unto me both in Jerusalem and in all Judea, and in Samaria, and unto the uttermost part of the earth" (Acts 1:8 UT).

"Rejoice always, pray without ceasing, in everything give thanks; for this is the will of God in Christ Jesus for you" (1 Thessalonians 5:16-18 NKJV).

"**Do not fret** because of evildoers, nor be envious of the workers of iniquity. For they shall soon be cut down like the grass, and wither as the green herb. **Trust** in the LORD, and do good; dwell in the land, and feed on His faithfulness. **Delight** yourself also in the LORD, and He shall give you the desires of your heart. **Commit** your way to the LORD, trust also in Him, and He shall bring it to pass. He shall bring forth your righteousness as the light, and your justice as the noonday. **Rest** in the LORD, and **wait** patiently for Him; **do not fret** because of him who prospers in his way, because of the man who brings wicked schemes to pass. **Cease** from anger, and forsake wrath; **do not fret**—it only causes harm. For evildoers shall be cut off; but those who **wait** on the LORD, they shall inherit the earth. For yet a little while and the wicked shall be no more; indeed, you will look diligently for his place, but it shall be no more. But the meek shall inherit the earth, and shall delight themselves in the abundance of peace" (Psalm 37:1-11 NKJV). (Trust – Delight – Commit – Rest – Wait)

"Even the youths shall faint and be weary, and the young men shall utterly fall, but they that **wait** on the LORD shall renew their strength; they shall mount up with wings like eagles, they shall run and not be weary, they shall walk and not faint" (Isaiah 40:30, 31 NKJV).

"Then Peter and the other apostles answered and said: We ought to obey God rather than men" (Acts 5:29 NKJV). See Joshua 24:14, 15.

"And let us consider one another in order to stir up love and good works, not forsaking the assembling of ourselves together, as is the manner of some, but exhorting one another, and so much the more as you see the Day approaching" (Hebrews 10:24, 25 NKJV).

Maintain a benevolent, thankful attitude toward God and others. Make a joyful noise unto the LORD, all you lands. Serve the LORD with gladness: come before His presence with singing. Know you that the LORD He is God: it is He that has made us, and not we ourselves; we are His people, and the sheep of His pasture. Enter into His gates with thanksgiving, and into His courts with praise; be thankful unto Him, and bless His name. For the LORD is good; His mercy is everlasting; and His truth endures to all generations (Psalm 100 UT). But the fruit of the Spirit is love, joy, peace, longsuffering, gentleness, goodness, faith, meekness, temperance: against such there is no law (Galatians 5:22, 23). See also 2 Timothy 2:15-26.

Love people in thought, word and deed. Let all bitterness, and wrath, and anger, and clamor, and evil speaking, be put away from you, with all malice: and be kind one to another, tenderhearted, forgiving one another, even as God for Christ's sake has forgiven you (Ephesians 4:31, 32 UT).

To have a good relationship with God, others and yourself, you must have a correct Christian theology! So, let us formulate a Christian theology.

FORMULATING A CHRISTIAN THEOLOGY

I. GOD

I believe that there is only one true and living God Who is worthy of my worship and service, that He as an Eternal Spirit is transcendent of His creation; infinite in all His attributes; omnipotent; omnipresent; omniscient; infinite in wisdom; perfect in goodness, mercy, love, justice and faithfulness; holy in His essential nature, attributes and purpose; and as Triune God in His essential being is revealed as Father, Son and Holy Spirit.

I believe God the Father is co-eternal, co-equal, consubstantial and has personal subsistence with the Son and the Holy Spirit.

I believe that God's providence is inherent in His sovereign will in maintaining the universe, that the miracles of God on earth are the laws of God in heaven, and that He does not violate the free moral agency of His created beings in things pertaining to their salvation and eternal destiny.

I stand opposed to **tritheism**, that there are three gods; **sabellianism**, that there is one God manifested in three relationships to the human race; **arianism**, that the Godhead consists of one eternal person, who in the beginning created a super-angelic being, the only begotten Son, who in turn created the Holy Spirit; **polytheism**, that there are many gods; **dualism**, that the universe is composed of two impersonal forces—mind and matter; and **pantheism**, that God and the universe are one and the

14

same.

Scriptures: Deuteronomy 4:35; 1 Kings 8:60; Psalm 86:9, 10; Isaiah 43:10, 11; John 17:3; Ephesians 4:6; Colossians 1:15; Genesis 21:33; Psalm 90:2; Revelation 4:8-11; Jeremiah 23:24; 2 Chronicles 6:18; Job 11:7-9; Psalm 147:5; Isaiah 40:28; Romans 11:33-36; Jeremiah 32:17; Revelation 19:6; Genesis 1:1; Psalm 33:13, 14; Jeremiah 23:23, 24; Isaiah 46:9, 10; Isaiah 40:12-15; Psalm 113:5-9; Daniel 2:20-22; Ephesians 1:7-9; Matthew 19:17; 1 Peter 1:16, 17; Jonah 3:4, 10; Psalm 104:4, 5; Matthew 3:13-17; Matthew 28:19; 2 Corinthians 13:14; Ephesians 2:18.

John 3:13; 6:32, 33, 38, 50, 51, 58, 62; John 1:1-3, 14; Hebrews 2:14-16; 1 Timothy 1:17; 6:16; Isaiah 9:6; Revelation 1:11; 2:8; 22:13; Matthew 28:20; John 2:24, 25; Galatians 2:3; Philippians 3:21; Hebrews 1:10-12; John 16:15; Colossians 2:9; Matthew 9:2-7; Galatians 3:13; Philippians 3:20, 21; Hebrews 1:6; Revelation 5:11, 12; Philippians 2:9-11; John 14:16, 17, 26; 15:26; 17:7, 14, 15; 1 Corinthians 2:10, 11; Acts 15:28; Acts 7:51; Isaiah 63:10; Ephesians 4:30; Matthew 12:31, 32; Acts 5:3, 4, 9; Genesis 6:3; John 16:13; Romans 8:26; 15:19; 1 Corinthians 6:11; Acts 13:2, 4; 1 Corinthians 12:11; Ephesians 1:13; 4:30; 2 Timothy 3:16; Isaiah 6:5, 9; Romans 8:26, 27; 1 Corinthians 2:10, 11; Romans 15:19; Titus 3:5; 2 Corinthians 13:14; Matthew 10:20; Galatians 4:6; Matthew 28:18; Ephesians 1:22; Hebrews 1:3; Revelation 17:14.

Job 9:5-8; Psalm 104:32; Matthew 5:45; Isaiah 40:12.

15

II. THE BIBLE

I believe the Bible is God's complete revelation of His will for the whole human race concerning our eternal salvation, as well as our duties and privileges in relation to His sovereign will for time and eternity, which could not be revealed by His material creation or human reasoning.

I believe that God's progressive revelation was completed within my present Bible of 39 books in the Old Testament and 27 books in the New Testament, so that whatever is not found written therein is not to be imposed as a doctrine or practice upon the Church of Jesus Christ.

I believe the Bible became the infallible Word of God, as God superintended the natural powers and faculties of holy men to write His Word without error. This is best explained in 2 Peter 1:20, 21.

I believe the purpose of the Bible is clearly stated in 2 Timothy 3:16, 17.

I believe in a literal interpretation of the Bible.

There was a flood, Jonah was swallowed by a great fish, Jesus was born of the virgin Mary, etc.

I stand opposed to any **further written or oral revelation** that is to bring new light to the Church or to the world. Furthermore, **I do not accept the apocryphal books** as a part of the Old Testament Scriptures. I stand opposed to all forms of criticism which do not accept the whole Bible as the Word of God.

Scriptures: 2 Peter 1:20, 21; 3:16; 2 Timothy 3:16, 17; Psalm 119; Matthew 2:23; John 6:45; Revelation 22:18, 19; Deuteronomy 4:2; 12:32; Proverbs 30:6; Exodus 32:33.

16

III. SPECIAL CREATION

I believe true science and a correct interpretation of the Bible are never in conflict with each other. The Bible acts as a supplement to the revealed truths of creation.

I believe special creation reveals the existence of God, His natural attributes, His works, and awakens me to a sense of accountability to Him.

I believe God, as my Creator and Redeemer, has the authority to command my loving service and complete obedience for time and eternity.

I believe the creation was planned by God the Father, brought forth by God the Son through God the Holy Spirit, as an act of His love and desire for fellowship and exultation.

I believe God created everything (material and spiritual) from nothing and formed them into the present creation as explained in Genesis 1 and 2 and Hebrews 11:3.

I stand opposed to **atheistic materialism**, which acts as though God does not exist and material is eternal; **pantheism**, which says matter is the eternal God; and all forms of **naturalistic progressive evolution**, which deny the plain teaching of God's Holy Word.

Scriptures: Gen. 1; 2; Hebrews 11:3; Psalm 19:1-6; 33:6; 148:5; John 9:17; Genesis 49:26; Job 38:4; Proverbs 8:22; John 1:1-3; Romans 1:20.

IV. ANGELS

I believe that angels are intelligent beings possessing great strength; are not able to reproduce their kind; have spiritual bodies; are incorruptible, immortal, and invisible; are not omnipotent, omnipresent, or omniscient; and that God created them as holy beings with the power to choose between good and evil.

I believe that a great number of the angels chose evil and plunged themselves into apostasy, torment, and damnation, and are organized totally against the plans and purposes of God.

I believe there is an actual devil, called Satan, who is the incarnation of evil, the avowed enemy of the human race, the leader of the wicked angels (demons) that fell in the beginning. Furthermore, he is the antichrist spirit, who is in the world today transforming himself into an angel of light to deceive people. He is limited in his wicked influences by the providence of God, and his end is eternal fire and brimstone in hell.

I believe people can be possessed (under complete control) by demons or oppressed (afflicted and tormented) by demons.

I believe that the holy angels are ministering spirits to the saints to:

      a. reveal God's will in special cases;

      b. preserve them from evil;

      c. convey their souls to heaven at death; and

      d. gather them together when they are raptured.

I believe that angels have revealed themselves to people in visible forms.

18

I stand opposed to any teaching, which states that angels are only impersonal good or evil principles or influences. I stand opposed to angels being worshiped.

Scriptures: 1 Corinthians 15:44; Genesis 18:2; 2 Peter 2:11; Psalm 103:20; 1 Peter 1:12; Matthew 22:30; Job 38:7; Hebrews 1:14; Jude 6; 1 Timothy 3:6; Ephesians 2:2; 6:12; Matthew 18:20; 2 Peter 2:4; Matthew 25:41; Matthew 13:39; John 8:44; Job 1; Ephesians 2:2; Revelation 20:7, 8; 2 Thessalonians 2:9, 10; 2 Corinthians 2:11; 1 Peter 5:8; 2 Samuel 14:17; Matthew 25:31; Daniel 10:13; 2 Kings 19:35; Psalm 91:10, 12; 34:7; Matthew 18:10; Luke 16:22; Revelation 19:10.

V. MANKIND

I believe that mankind in his original state was created with a threefold nature of body (which was of the dust of the earth), soul (which is our life energy), and spirit (which was created in God's image and likeness), possessing the attributes of being spiritual, social, creative, a free moral agent, rational, holy and immortal; had a complete and unbroken communion with his Creator God; was created as a finite being a little lower than the angels; and was placed in the Garden of Eden (a land of perfect happiness), to rule the earth, to reproduce their kind, and to grow in the grace and knowledge of the Lord.

I believe that Adam, as the representative of mankind, was created first; that Eve was created from a rib of Adam; and these two were the common parents of the whole human race.

19

I believe that when Adam fell from his original state by an act of disobedience, he died spiritually; the image of God in mankind was defaced; he became totally depraved, and plunged the whole human race into sin with all its consequences.

I believe mankind as a free moral agent, who is able to know right from wrong, can freely choose the moral path he will take.

I believe mankind is unable to save himself from sin.

I believe mankind can be restored to moral purity in this life through the blood of Jesus Christ.

I believe God has provided a complete restoration for the whole human race through the blood atonement of Jesus, which must be accepted on an individual basis.

I stand opposed to **rationalism**, which says the rational part of man was not affected by the fall and makes reason the sole source of knowledge for actions; **gnosticism**, which says the spirit of man is an emanation from God and thus makes me a little god; and **socialism**, which denies depravity in the human race, and makes injustices within the social environment the cause of moral depravity.

Scriptures: Genesis 1-3; Psalm 8; Genesis 5:3; 6; Genesis 3:15; John 3:16; 2 Peter 3:9; Isaiah 53.

VI. SIN

I believe sin is twofold in nature, in that it is a willful transgression against a known law of God, and an inherited proneness toward evil, which corrupts the whole human nature.

I believe this corruption of human nature remains in the born-again child of God until it is eradicated by the infilling of the Holy Spirit at sanctification.

I believe the effect of sin is total depravity to the extent that without a Redeemer I would be hopelessly and eternally lost.

I believe sin is in the world because of Adam's fall and man's own willful rebellion against God.

I believe the penalty of sin is both physical and spiritual death.

I believe God's attitude toward sin is present wrath and eternal vengeance on the sinner who refuses to repent.

I believe everyone is a sinner by birth and by choice until Jesus becomes His Saviour and Lord.

I stand opposed to any teaching that denies the utter sinfulness of the whole human race.

Scriptures: Genesis 3; 5:3; 6:5; Psalm 10:2-11; 51:5; Jeremiah 17:9; Romans 3; 6:23; Ezekiel 18:20-23; John 3:36; 1 Corinthians 3:1-3.

VII. THE JEWISH NATION

I believe the Jews are God's chosen people to bring the Redeemer of mankind and His earthly kingdom into the world.

I believe the Old Testament Scriptures show God's dealings with the Jewish people.

I believe the promises God has given to the Jews are literal and will be literally fulfilled.

Scriptures: Isaiah 51:2; Deuteronomy 7:6, 7; 14:2; Exodus 19:5, 6; Deuteronomy 32:10, 11; 33:27-29; Psalm 105:13-15; Psalm 121:3-5; Genesis 49:10; Daniel 9:25; Psalm 14:7; Romans 11:26; Ezekiel 39:29; Zechariah 12:10; Romans 11:25; Hosea 3:5; Isaiah 44:22; 59:20; Jeremiah 33:8; Isaiah 44:23; 49:13; 52:8, 9; 66:10, 19; Jeremiah 3:18; Isaiah 11:15, 16; 14:1-3; 49:22, 23; 60:11, 12, 14, 19; 61:4-6; Isaiah 59:20; Zechariah 2:11; Romans 11:24.

VIII. SALVATION

I believe that Jesus Christ (Who was born of the Virgin Mary), lived a life without sin, died on a cross, was buried in a tomb, rose the third day, revealed Himself alive in a resurrected body by many infallible proofs for 40 days, ascended into heaven having obtained eternal redemption for me, and is now seated on the right hand of God the Father, interceding for me. He is perfect God and perfect man—the God-man. I believe Jesus will come again to put away wickedness and set up His kingdom upon this earth.

I believe Jesus is the only provision for my eternal redemption.

I believe salvation is threefold:

a. I am saved from the guilt of sin when I repent of my sins and accept Jesus as my own personal Savior by faith.

b. I am saved from the power of sin when I fully consecrate myself to God and by faith accept the Holy Spirit as my Sanctifier after I am saved.

c. I am saved from the effects of sin, either when I die a Christian or I am raptured into glory at the second coming of Jesus Christ.

I believe salvation is received by faith in God's finished work, which is through Jesus Christ.

I believe salvation is personal and knowable.

I believe salvation is for the whole person for time and eternity.

I believe "saved," "eternal redemption," "regeneration," "born-again," "conversion" are all expressions showing a new life through faith in the shed blood of Jesus Christ.

I believe "atonement," "justification," "reconciliation," "propitiation" are expressions showing God's mercy in forgiving my sins and freeing me from its guilt and penalty when I repent of my sins and accept Jesus as my Savior.

I believe adoption is that gracious act of God whereby I am made a child of God.

I believe eternal life is God's gift to me when I become a child of God.

I believe I receive regeneration, justification, adoption and eternal life in the first definite work of God's grace. I believe I receive the Holy Spirit at this time. I believe the original sin remains in a subdued condition in this first work of God's grace.

I believe "original sin," "selfishness," "the old man," "carnality," "the flesh," "the body of sin," "the law of sin and death," "the body of death," "the besetting sin," "the sin of the world" are all expressions of the inherited depravity of my moral nature by which I am led into sin from birth to sanctification, at which time this nature is purged out.

I believe entire sanctification is a second definite work of God's grace by which God cleanses His adopted child from the inner defilement of his human nature. I believe when I give my life completely to God and trust Him for His cleansing, I am filled with the Holy Spirit. I believe entire sanctification brings me into a life of holy living.

I believe "holiness," "Christian holiness," "Christian perfection," "perfect love," "perfect peace," "heart holiness," "rest of faith" are all expressions of a life of love, which can only be lived as the Holy Spirit sheds the love of God abroad in my heart.

I believe the life of holiness is progressive in that I grow in the grace and knowledge of my Lord and Savior, Jesus Christ all my Christian life.

I stand opposed to: **baptismal regeneration**, which states a person is born again into God's family when baptized in water with the baptismal formula; a **limited atonement**, which states God has elected some to be saved and some to be lost, or that you have to fight the carnal spirit all your Christian life; a **works salvation**, which says I am saved by works or receive grace through the good works of others; and **unconditional eternal security**, which says once I am saved I never can backslide and be eternally lost in hell.

Scripture: Isaiah 7:14; Matthew 1:18-23; Hebrews 4:15; Matthew 27:50, 58-60; 28:5-10; Acts 1:3-11; 1 Corinthians 15:3-8; Hebrews 7:25; 9:12; 1 Timothy 3:16; Matthew 25:31-46; Revelation 20:11-15; John 14:6; Acts 4:12; Romans 5; 6; 1 Corinthians 15; Romans 5:1; Ephesians 2:8-10; John 3:16; Acts 15:8, 9; John 3:1-3; Romans 8:14-21; Hebrews 10:14, 15; 1 John 5:18-21; Romans 8 with 1:8; 1 Thessalonians 1 with 4:3-8; 5:23, 24; John 7:37-39; Acts 8:14-17; 19:1-7; Romans 5:5; 2 Corinthians 7:11. Galatians 2:20; 4:4-6; 5:16-26; 6:7-9,14-16; 2 Peter 1:1-9;

24

3:18.

IX. THE CHRISTIAN MINISTRY

I believe in a God-inspired, God-called, and God-equipped Christian ministry.

I believe that both men and women are called into the Christian ministry to preach God's Word and pastor a church.

I believe the extent of the Christian ministry is for each organized church, for all cultures, for all time.

I believe the purpose of the Christian ministry is to propagate the gospel of Jesus Christ to the ends of the world, to organize new churches, and to administer the laws, sacraments, and disciplines of the church.

I believe the Christian ministry is equipped spiritually, mentally, emotionally, and socially through personal experience and training.

I believe the Christian minister should know the gospel, live the gospel, be gentle to the contentious, and be apt to teach and ready to preach the gospel to others individually and collectively.

I believe only those who meet the qualifications, as set forth in 1 and 2 Timothy and Titus, should be allowed to preach or teach in the church.

I believe every Christian has a called ministry, whether it is being a good parent or pastoring a church. I believe the gifts of the Spirit are given to Christians to minister to, and for the advancement of, God's kingdom upon the earth through the Church of Jesus Christ my Lord and Saviour.

I stand opposed to an **unprepared ministry**, which

25

allows one to minister without showing Biblical qualifications for it; a **liberal ministry**, which rejects the literal and authoritative nature of the Word of God; **an elite ministry**, which states only the pastor can witness for Christ and have a full understanding of the deep things of God; and a **social ministry**, which places social issues above spiritual issues and denies my need of a born-again experience within the church membership.

Scriptures: 1 and 2 Timothy; Titus; 1 Thessalonians 5:12, 13; Matthew 26:18-20; Acts 1:8; 2:17, 18; Romans 10:11-17; 1 Corinthians 12.

X. THE CHRISTIAN CHURCH

I believe the true Christian Church consists of all true "called-out" followers of God in all generations who have organized themselves together to propagate the gospel of Christ to the uttermost parts of the earth.

I believe the purpose of the Christian Church is to provide Christian worship, Christian fellowship, a Christian ministry, and a Christian witness for every born-again child of God.

I believe the true Christian Church is separated from the world by the mighty working of the Holy Spirit, with the purpose of pointing the unregenerate world to a better way of life.

I believe Jesus is the head of the Church, which is the body of Christ.

I believe the power of the Christian Church is through the moral purity and inspiration it receives from the indwelling

Holy Spirit.

I believe the purity of the Christian Church covers three areas:

a. not conformed to the world,

b. freed from the carnal nature, and

c. not bound by evil influences of satanic powers.

I believe this purity makes the Christian Church free to follow God completely in all things.

I believe the Church has the right and obligation to discipline its members.

I believe the Church has two sacraments, baptism and the Lord's Supper, which were instituted by Jesus for all generations.

I believe the financial needs of the Christian Church should be met by tithes and offerings.

I stand opposed to a **one-church salvation**, which states I have to be a member of their church to get to heaven; a **formalized worship**, which leaves no place for God to work in a church service to bring a sinner to a personal faith in Christ; **consubstantiation or transubstantiation**, which states the body and blood of Christ is with, or becomes one with the elements of the Lord's supper, respectively; **denominationalism**, which places dogma and traditions above the plain teachings of the Bible.

Scriptures: Matthew 16:18; 18:17-20; Acts 2:47; 5:11; 7:38; 14:23; 20:28; 1 Corinthians 4:17; 11:20-30; 12:28; 14:5, 33; Ephesians 5:23-32; Colossians 1:18, 24; 1 Timothy 3:5, 15, 16; Hebrews 12:23; James 5:14; Matthew 26:26-30; Luke 14:22-26; Luke 22:14-20; Matthew 28:19.

XI. THE CIVIL GOVERNMENT

I believe the laws of the civil government are instituted by God and that I am to obey them, so long as they do not violate my God-given freedoms of worshiping and witnessing for Him.

I believe the purpose of the civil government is to secure my God-given rights to life, liberty, and the pursuit of happiness as stated in the Declaration of Independence, July 4, 1776.

I believe the civil government has a right to finance its constitutional obligations to its citizens through fair and representative taxation.

I believe the civil government is to administer protection and justice to its people, the Church is to minister to the spiritual needs of the people, and that the two are not to interfere with each other's God-given duties.

I stand opposed to the **civil government regulating the Christian Church**; to a **State Elite Church**, which sanctions only one denomination as the Official Church that can function within its citizenship; and to **Atheistic Socialism**, which wants to remove everything that has to do with God and the Church out of my governmental and public institutions.

Scriptures: Acts 4:19, 20; 5:29; Romans 13; 1 Peter 3:22; Psalm 9:17.

XII. THE WORLD

I believe "the world" is the unregenerate segment of my society, under the control of Satan, working as a substitute for real Christianity.

I believe the Christian is to be separated from worldly pleasures (dancing, ungodly movies and TV, drug addiction, loose living), worldly fads (religious fads, indecent dress), and worldly attitudes (rebellion, party spirit). As a Christian, I am in the world, but not a part of its ungodly system.

Scriptures: Romans 12:1, 2; 2 Corinthians 4:4; Galatians 1:4; Titus 2:12; Matthew 5:14; 16:26; John 1:10-13, 29; John 4:42; 14:17; 15:19; 16:8- 11, 33; 17:14, 16, 21; Romans 3:19; 1 Corinthians 1:2; 2:12; 3:19; 5:10; Galatians 6:14; Ephesians 2:2; Philippians 2:15; 1 Timothy 1:15; James 1:27; 4:4; 2 Peter 1:4; 2:20; 1 John 2:15-17; 3:1; 5:4, 5, 19; Revelation 11:15; Deuteronomy 22:5; 1 Timothy 2:9, 10; 1 Peter 3:3, 4.

In our next prescription we are going to show how to remove enemies of ultimate health. The special note gets us to thinking about a new approach to maintaining good health.

Special Note

Everything done by the medical profession can be done much better with natural remedies without the side effects!

29

PRESCRIPTION 2 - ELIMINATE ENEMIES OF ULTIMATE HEALTH

Remove all resentments from your life by loving God and others. "Who is a wise man and endued with knowledge among you? Let him show out of a good conversation (conduct) his works with meekness of wisdom. But if you have bitter envying and strife in your hearts, glory not, and lie not against the truth. This wisdom descends not from above, but is earthly, sensual, devilish. For where envying and strife is, there is confusion and every evil work. But the wisdom that is from above is first pure, then peaceable, gentle, and easy to be entreated, full of mercy and good fruits, without partiality, and without hypocrisy. And the fruit of righteousness is sown in peace of them that make peace" (James 3:13-18 UT).

Remove stress from your life by casting all your cares on Him. "Be careful for nothing; but in everything by prayer and supplication with thanksgiving let your requests be made known unto God. And the peace of God, which passes all understanding, shall keep your hearts and minds through Christ Jesus. Finally, brothers whatsoever things are true, whatsoever things are honest, whatsoever things are just, whatsoever things are pure, whatsoever things are lovely, whatsoever things are of good report; if there be any virtue, and if there be any praise, think on these things" (Philippians 4:6-8). "Casting all your care upon Him; for He cares for you (1 Peter 5:7 UT).

Slowly remove all processed and cooked foods from your diet. These foods are packed full of harmful poisons that overwork your immune system. As stated earlier, you need to maintain a Ph of 7.4 in your body. Animal flesh is very acidic. If the food is too acidic, your body will leach out the calcium from your bones. Cow's milk is for baby cows. You cannot improve on an all-raw organic diet of fruits, vegetables, nuts, seeds, herbs and spices. Soak the seeds to release their energy benefits. You do not need protein. You need amino acids so your body can make its own protein. You do not need to count calories. You need to think of enzymes, which are the live part of the foods you eat.

Much research has gone into the causes of disease in the "civilized" nations. The Price-Pottenger Nutritional Foundation has pioneered work done by two men. Price compared our diet to the native diet. Pottenger did experiments using cats. This foundation has developed "Guidelines For Good Health." The American Institute For Cancer Research has come to a similar conclusion in their research. They have developed a "Foods That Fight Cancer" directive. These organizations do allow for some meats in their diets. It should be noted that these organizations place limitations on meat consumption.

I do not agree with all their "findings." As you will see later in this book I am suggesting an all-raw-organic diet that eliminates all animal products. More on this later.

Make sure all body and spiritual wastes are removed regularly and completely.

This will be automatic if you are doing the things listed in this book. When your body tells you to go, do what it is prompting you to do. Do not put it off. This will only mess up your regular cycle.

The other thing that you need to do is remove spiritual

31

waste. This has to do with doctrines that are against the plain teachings of the Judeo-Christian Bible. Anything that hinders your spiritual growth in God's love and grace is a spiritual waste. If you let these things accumulate in your spiritual life they will destroy your relationships with God and others. Anything that causes your devotional life to grow cold is a spiritual waste. If there is a strained relationship with others it is a spiritual waste.

Here are some Scriptures that will help you remove spiritual waste from your life:

"Keep your tongue from evil, and your lips from speaking guile. Depart from evil, and do good; seek peace, and pursue it (Psalm 34:13, 14 NKJV).

"You rebuke the proud—the cursed, who stray from Your commandments. Remove from me reproach and contempt, for I kept Your testimonies" (Psalm 119:21, 22 NKJV).

"Remove from me the way of lying, and grant me Your law graciously" (Psalm 119:29 NKJV).

"Do not turn to the right or the left; Remove your foot from evil" (Proverbs 4:27 NKJV).

"For the lips of an immoral woman drip honey, and her mouth is smoother than oil; but in the end she is bitter as wormwood, sharp as a two-edged sword. . . . Remove your way far from her, and do not go near her house, lest you give your honor to others, and your labors go to the house of foreigners; and you mourn at last, when your flesh and your body are consumed, and say: How I have hated instruction, and my heart despised reproof!" (Proverbs 5:3, 4, 8-12 NKJV).

"Do you not know that your bodies are members of Christ? Shall I then take the members of Christ and make

32

them members of a harlot? Certainly not! Or do you not know that he who is joined to a harlot is one body with her? For the two, he says, shall become one flesh. But he who is joined to the Lord is one spirit with Him. Flee sexual immorality. Every sin that a man does is outside the body, but he who commits sexual immorality sins against his own body" (1 Corinthians 6:15-18 NKJV).

"Remove falsehood and lies far from me; give me neither poverty nor riches—feed me with the food You prescribe for me; lest I be full and deny You, and say, Who is the LORD? Or lest I be poor and steal, and profane the name of my God (Proverbs 30:8, 9 NKJV).

PRESCRIPTION 3 - GATHER FRIENDS OF ULTIMATE HEALTH

Eat an all-raw diet of organic fruits, vegetables, seeds, nuts, spices and herbs. "And God said, Behold, I have given you every herb bearing seed, which is upon the face of all the earth, and every tree, in the which is the fruit of a tree yielding seed; to you it shall be for meat (food)" (Genesis 1:29).

It is important that you eat your food raw and that it be free of all added substances like additives and preservatives. The ideal would be for you to have your own organic garden. You should sprout your seeds. Never heat any of your food above 107° F.

I used to think food must be cooked to digest properly. This is not true. My wife and I have been on a raw food diet for over 10 years. We have no problems with digestion. We have learned when we do not cook our food we do not need to eat as much. Why is this? Cooked food is dead food. Raw food is live food. We are both in our 70's without many of the sicknesses that plague our society. We are doing very well physically and spiritually.

This is something to think about. Before meat was introduced into the human diet people lived much longer. After meat was introduced into the human diet people lived shorter lives. Before the flood people lived on an average of 912 years. After the flood the average ages decreased with each generation—from 900's to 600's to 400's to 200's to 100's. By the time you get to David's generation the average age is between 70 and 80. Before the flood people

34

were not plagued with the diseases we have today. After the flood, diseases have plagued the human race. There are two possible reasons for this. One, the earth was not the same as before the flood. This is an unlikely reason because of the fact that people did live to be over 600 years old after the flood. Two, meat and cooked food does something to our immune system. This picture looks much like what Doctors Price and Pottenger discovered in their research. The good news is that when Pottenger put his sick/deformed cats on a good diet each generation improved. This would be a good reason for anyone who longs for better health to take heed to what is put forth in this book. Take a look at the research that is referenced below. The *American Institute For Cancer Research* has some very helpful information on its website. This is also referenced below. You may also want to check out my research that I did on the Ezine Articles website. The links are listed at the end of this book on the "Further Studies" page.

Daily drink one ounce of pure distilled water per two pounds of body weight. This is a minimum amount—more in hot weather. Your body is over 70 percent water and your brain is more like 80 percent. Make sure you do not get dehydrated. It is very important for you to get pure water. Your best source of pure water is organic vegetable and fruit juices. Norman W. Walker's book, *Fresh Vegetable and Fruit Juices*, shows how juicing can greatly improve your health using vegetable and fruit juices.

Some things you will need for this diet are: a high quality juicer (such as Green Star or Champion), food processor, a dehydrator with a temperature-control (most foods dry well at 105 to 107 degrees), a good water distiller and high-powered blender. You will also need a good cutting board and some good, sharp knives. You will need some measuring cups and spoons. In bigger cities you may be able to find a support group you can get with to learn more about this diet. There are several websites you can log onto that will help you.

It may surprise you to know you can make such things as breads, cakes, pies, pizzas, nutritious salads, soups, ice cream, smoothies, health-enhancing juice mixtures, etc. using this diet. There are helpful recipes in this book!

There is a much greater variety of foods you can eat when you eat an all-raw diet of fruits, vegetables, nuts, seeds, spices and herbs. There are endless combinations of dishes that can be made. Also, you will find there are some foods you should not mix. The rule is, keep it simple.

Try to buy organic produce as much as possible. If not available, or not in your price range, be sure to wash your food with a good organic wash before you eat or prepare it. Rinse well before using. (Much of the food can be eaten as is). (Strawberries, broccoli and pineapple are the exception to using a wash and should just be rinsed in cool water (distilled, if possible).

There are some outstanding testimonies of people who have been healed from all kinds of diseases by using this diet. Also, my experience has been, the longer I stay on this diet the healthier I become. However, this diet is not a miracle cure for every physical or emotional problem. There are limits. Just because others have had outstanding results using this diet does not mean you will. When you are in the detoxing stage, when you first go on this diet you may have some discomfort such as aches, pains, headaches, turning yellow, weight loss, possible diarrhea and feeling faint. As you stay on the diet these symptoms will go away. Your body will reach equilibrium and you will experience much better health. If you experience some of the above symptoms, make the transfer from old to new more slowly. Also, during the detox stage, drink an extra amount of vegetable and fruit juices and distilled water. This will help your body remove the toxins. At this stage you will also be removing more body waste. This is another reason why you need to drink more liquids. Otherwise, you could get dehydrated.

You do not need to eat animal flesh to get your protein. This diet supplies all the nutrients you will need. I do take a vitamin B12 supplement, but this can be covered with nutritional yeast. You should use unheated sea salt and natural sugars like honey, raisins, dates, figs or stevia.

If you cannot get organic foods, you will need to make sure you get the freshest ones, preferably from farmers' markets, that are not waxed (or dried fruits that are not sulfured). Some foods will need to be purchased at a health food store. Stay away from all additives, processed and artificial food products. This is especially true for artificial sweeteners. Nitrates and nitrites should also be eliminated from your diet. Check labels before you buy a canned, packaged or bottled product.

PRESCRIPTION 4 - KEEP A REGULAR SCHEDULE

Develop a daily regular scheduled time for food, rest, devotions and exercise. Your body has a biological clock. It likes to do things in a regular, orderly fashion. Your biological clock works on a day/night cycle. You can reset it within limits.

Your body knows what it needs. For example, you need to be out in the sunshine for good health. This is the reason a person feels depressed on a cloudy day. If you will listen to your body, it will tell you what it needs.

Food should be taken 2 or 3 times a day. Do not eat too much at a time. The big meal should be taken in the middle of the day. Water should be taken throughout the day according to your body weight—one ounce of water for every 2 pounds of body weight. More in hot weather. When you are thirsty or feel like you have the flu, drink more water and/or juices.

Rest should be taken no later than 10:00 PM for those who are working hard throughout the day. When you are tired, go to bed. This is your body's way of saying it is rest time.

Devotions should be at the start and end of your day. There should be private and family devotions. Get a good devotional book and use it. Let everyone participate in the family devotions. This is a good time to help each other with problems that may arise. Also, this is a good time to share each other's blessings and insights the Lord has given. Make this time the best time of your day.

Your exercise program should be fitted into your schedule. Morning is usually the best time to have your exercise. You may have to join an exercise club. Perhaps you can walk in the park or around a few blocks. Be creative with this one.

Whatever schedule you choose, keep with it. If you have something unexpected come up, just tend to it and get back on schedule as soon as possible. This will take some self discipline.

"To everything there is a season, a time for every purpose under heaven: a time to be born, and a time to die; a time to plant, and a time to pluck up what is planted; a time to kill and a time to heal; a time to break down, and a time to build up; a time to weep, and a time to laugh; a time to mourn, and a time to dance; a time to cast away stones, and a time to gather stones: a time to embrace, and a time to refrain from embracing; a time to gain, and a time to lose; a time to keep, and a time to throw away; a time to tear, and a time to sew; a time to keep silent, and a time to speak; a time to love, and a time to hate; a time of war, and a time of peace. . . . He has made everything beautiful in its time" (Ecclesiastes 3:1-8, 11a NKJV).

"See then that you walk circumspectly, not as fools but as wise, redeeming the time, because the days are evil. Therefore do not be unwise, but understand what the will of the Lord is" (Ephesians 5:15-17 NKJV).

PRESCRIPTION 5 - PERFECT REST

Get at least eight hours of rest a day. Rest more in stressful times. You must give yourself proper rest so your body and mind can rejuvenate itself. "It is vain for you to rise up early, to sit up late, to eat the bread of sorrows: for so He gives His beloved sleep" (Psalm 127:2 UT).

Rest with a good conscience at the end of the day. "Now the end of the commandment is charity (self-giving love), out of a pure heart, and a good conscience, and of faith unfeigned (without pretense)" (1 Timothy 1:7).

"For, if you forgive men their trespasses, your Heavenly Father will also forgive you. But, if you forgive not men their trespasses, neither will your Father forgive your trespasses" (Matthew 6:14, 15 UT).

"Be angry and sin not, let not the sun go down upon your wrath: Neither give place to the devil" (Ephesians 4:26, 27 UT).

"Now the **works of the flesh** are manifest, which are: adultery, fornication, uncleanness, lasciviousness, Idolatry, witchcraft, hatred, variance, emulations, wrath, strife, seditions, heresies, Envyings, murders, drunkenness, revelings, and such like: of the which I told you before, as I have told you in time past, that they which do such things shall not inherit the kingdom of God. But the **fruit of the Spirit** is love, joy, peace, longsuffering, gentleness, goodness, faith, Meekness, temperance: against such there is no law. And they that are Christ's, have crucified the flesh with its affections and lusts. If we live in the Spirit, let us also walk in the Spirit. Let us not be desirous of vain glory, provoking one another, envying one another" (Galatians 5:19-26 UT).

If you live an ungodly lifestyle, evidenced by living out the works of the flesh, your conscience will not allow you to rest. If you live for God, evidenced by living out the fruit of the Holy Spirit, you will be able to rest in God's love and grace.

If you have not lived right, get yourself right with God and others before you go to sleep. If you have been living a life pleasing to God, you can rest assured that everything is alright with your soul.

PRESCRIPTION 6 - ALL-INCLUSIVE EXERCISE

Exercise with a Rebounder or have a good walking program. The only way you can keep your immune system healthy is through physical exercise. The Rebounder may be purchased from:

> Needak Manufacturing, LLC
> Website: http://www.NeedakRebounders.com.
> Telephone: (800) 232-5762.

As you are doing your exercise you can do it with Christian music. This is a good way to express your faith and love to your Lord and Savior.

Exercise your faith and obedience toward God.

Recipe For Victorious Christian Living From Psalm 37

+FRET NOT yourself because of evil doers, neither be
 envious against the workers of iniquity.
+TRUST IN THE LORD and do good.
+DELIGHT YOURSELF IN THE LORD.
+COMMIT YOUR WAYS TO THE LORD.
+REST IN THE LORD.
+WAIT PATIENTLY FOR THE LORD.
+CEASE FROM ANGER, AND FORSAKE WRATH.
+FRET NOT YOURSELF IN ANY WISE TO DO EVIL.

Exercising your faith includes witnessing for the Lord. Tell others what the Lord has done for you. Live a life before people that shows them you love them as well as God. Be ready at all times to answer people's questions concerning your new life in Christ Jesus. Do not be

42

ashamed of the Lord and His Word. Trust God to help you "speak the truth in love." Do not be a "know-it-all." Show forth a meek and quiet spirit when talking to others concerning your faith. Share what God has done for you and your family.

PRESCRIPTION 7 - ENJOY GOD'S CREATION

Get some sunlight once or twice a day. Sunlight is very helpful for your health. Do not overdo a good thing. You can "kill three birds with one stone" by taking a walk outside in a place that has an abundance of plant life. This way you would get your exercise, sunlight and fresh air in its most natural form.

Breathe fresh air as much as possible. Fresh air is very important. You must have fresh oxygen and nitrogen from the air you breathe, as well as the foods you eat. Ninety-six percent (96%) of your nutrition comes from the air you breathe. Four percent (4%) comes from the food you eat. You can do without food for days, but you must have fresh air every moment of your life.

Work for the good of your family and those around you. God has created you for work. You are not to sit around all day and draw a check from the government if you are able to work. The government should not take from the rich to give to the poor. When the government takes from one group to support another one, they are committing robbery. If you are unable to work, then it is the duty of God's people to take care of you. However, the Church is under no obligation to take care of greedy or lazy people. In this case if you do not work, you do not eat. Taking care of the poor is to be voluntary according to people's ability to do so. It is the responsibility of each person who is able to do so, to take care of orphans and widows. Every church should have a relief program for the truly needy.

"Then the LORD God took the man and put him in the

44

garden of Eden to tend and keep it" (Genesis 2:15 NKJV). Later on He created a woman, whom Adam called Eve.

Genesis 1 and 2 show how God worked in creating the universe and a garden for our first parents. "Thus the heavens and the earth, and all the host of them, were finished. And on the seventh day God ended His work which He had done, and He rested on the seventh day from all His work which He had done. Then God blessed the seventh day and sanctified it, because in it He rested from all His work which God had created and made" (Genesis 2:1-3 NKJV).

"Man goes out to his work and to his labor until the evening" (Psalm 104:23 NKJV).

"Unless the LORD builds the house, they labor in vain who build it; unless the LORD guards the city, the watchman stays awake in vain" (Psalm 127:1 NKJV).

"The labor of the righteous leads to life, the wages of the wicked to sin" (Proverbs 10:16 NKJV. "The wages of sin is death, but the gift of God is eternal life in Christ Jesus our Lord" (Romans 6:23).

"The desire of the slothful (lazy) kills him, for his hands refuse to labor. He covets greedily all day long, but the righteous gives and does not spare" (Proverbs 21:25, 26 NKJV).

"For even when we were with you, we commanded you this: If anyone will not work, neither shall he eat." (2 Thessalonians 3:10).

CONCLUSION

If you follow these seven (7) prescriptions with their ingredients listed above, you will maintain a strong, healthy immune system, which will enable you to enjoy maximum health. You will not need to go to your doctor so he can drug, cut, or burn you back to "health." You cannot improve on God's program of good health. This is a whole new way of dealing with disease. If you do these things consistently, you will be free from many of the diseases that plague most people today. There are several helpful books, videos and other study aids listed at the end of this book.

COMBINING FOODS

Because different foods digest at different times in the stomach, it is important to understand digestion times for various foods. Not observing these times can result in stomach cramps.

Melons have less digestion times (between 15-30 minutes) so it's best not to combine any other fruit with them. But various types of melons may be combined.

Acid and Sub-Acid Fruits digest in approximately 1-1½ hrs. These are: sour and sweet apples (apple juice can be combined with carrot juice) sour and sweet cherries, cranberries, grapefruit, sour and sweet grapes, kiwis, kumquats, lemons (lemons and lemon juice combine well with all foods), limes, oranges, pineapples, sour and sweet plums, pomegranates, raspberries, star fruit, tangerines, most berries, cherimoya, fresh figs, guavas, mangoes, nectarines, papaya, peaches and pears.

Starches, Low-Starch Vegetables, Non-Starch Vegetables, and Fruit Vegetables digest in approximately 2-3 hrs. These are: all squashes, dried legumes, peas and beans, all flours, grains, potatoes, sweet potatoes, yams; beets, carrots, celeriac, corn, Jerusalem artichokes, parsnips, peas, rutabagas, turnips; all sprouts, all leaf lettuces, all sprouted greens, all greens, (not carrot) all cabbages, asparagus, bok choy, broccoli, cauliflower, celery, cilantro, zucchini, cucumbers, daicon radish, edible weeds, fennel, fresh herbs, green beans, jicama, kohlrabi, leeks, onions, red, yellow and orange bell peppers, radishes, scallions, watercress; tomatoes.

47

Sweet Fruits digest in approximately 3-4 hrs. These consist of all dried fruits, bananas, dates, persimmons, sapote.

Proteins digest in approximately 4 hrs. These consist of all beans, all nuts and nut-based dishes, all seeds and seed-based dishes, green coconuts, legumes, all soaked and sprouted nuts and seeds, all sprouted grains, peas and beans.

Avocados digest in 2¾ hrs. and combine well with all foods except proteins. NOTE: For those fighting cancer, avocados and all fat should be avoided. Fat feeds cancer.

HERBS THAT HEAL

There are a number of websites that list herbs that heal. Every disease healed by medical drugs can be healed with herbals without the side effects. My suggestion is www.healthherbs.com. The owner of Health Herbs is a Christian Master Herbalist with years of experience. He does free consultations over the phone. He has a free pdf download of herbs with extensive information about them. He manufactures herbal remedy products.

Materials For Further Studies Toward Immune System Health

Dr. Lorraine Day, MD. *Video Series*, Rockford Press, P. O. Box 8, Thousand Palms CA 92276, Telephone: 1-800-574-2436.

Dr. Norman W. Walker D. Sc., Norwalk Press, P. O. Box 12260, Prescott AZ 86304.

Dr. George H. Malkmus. *Why Christians Get Sick*, and others; Treasure House, P. O. Box 310, Shippensburg PA 17257.

The Cancer Answer by Albert E. Carter, Telephone: 1-800-232-5762.

There are many books on food preparation you can find in your health store. The authors listed above give several references for further study.

The American Institute For Cancer Research at www.aicr.org/foods-that-fight-cancer

Price-Pottenger Nutritional Foundation at www.ppnf.org/resources/guidelines-for-good-health

The author's articles at ezinearticles.com: www.ezinearticles.com/Finding-An-Alternative-Health-Program-That-Brings-Lasting-Health?&id=6101784 and www.ezinearticles.com/Can-an-Organic-Raw-Foods-Diet-Prevent-Cancer-and-Heart-Diseases?&id=6065720

RAW FOOD RECIPES

The nice thing about raw food recipes is, you can be creative. It is hard to do it wrong. I will give you some examples from *Arlene's Kitchen* and you can take it from there.

Here are some things to observe when preparing raw food recipes: (1) Eat melons by themselves. (2) Use as many vegetables as you can in your vegetable salads. (3) You can make your own sprouts from a number of different seeds. (4) Make sure the foods are a good quality. (5) Eat your big meal at noon. (6) Use first cold-pressed, extra virgin olive oil as well as avocados for your healthy oils. (7) Try to buy organic produce as much as possible. If not available, or not in your price range, wash your fruits and vegetables with a good food wash before preparing. (Strawberries, broccoli. pineapple and cantaloupe are the exception. Just rinse in cool water, distilled if possible). (8) Blend nuts and seeds with water in a high speed blender for "milk." (9) Drink as many juices as you are able. (10) Use herbs and spices to enhance your immune system. (11) Use a good dehydrator with a temperature control, rather than cooking your food. Do not heat your food above 105 to 107° F. (12) Drink distilled water. (13) Go from cooked foods to raw foods in stages as stated above. (14) Use natural salts like Celtic Sea Salt or Himalayan Pink Crystal Salt. (15) Use natural sweeteners like honey, agave, maple syrup, raisins, dates, figs or stevia. (16) Some ingredients will need to be purchased at a health food store.

The Hallelujah Diet allows 15% - 25% cooked food (at the end of the day) for those who cannot adhere to a strict raw food diet. Their website is www.hacres.com).

Another good website is www.rawfoodrecipes.com.

The following are just a few of our favorite simple recipes, intended for two people. There are many more which are more elaborate, adapted from books put out by chefs of raw food restaurants.

BREAKFAST

You can eat some raw fruit. This can be any that is in season. Make sure the fruit is ripe and clear of waxes before you eat it. Eat until you are satisfied.

Have a smoothie made of bananas, fresh blueberries, and nut milk.

Eat a few nuts, pumpkin seeds or some dates. **You can be creative with this!**

The following recipes are from Arlene's Kitchen.

Carrot Juice

3 lbs. Organic carrots, scrubbed (peeled, if not organic).
2 Gala, Pink Lady, or Jonathan apples "   "   "   "
   seeds removed
2 celery stalks
4 fresh beet leaves
2 thin slices of ginger root
4 stem ends cut from romaine lettuce (if you have)

In a heavy-duty juicer, process the above ingredients. If you are saving the carrot pulp for another recipe, juice the carrots first and collect the pulp in a container. If not, you may alternate the ingredients. This recipe should make four 8 oz. servings.

We have one serving apiece for breakfast. I store the other 2 servings in two 8 oz. canning jars for the next day's breakfast. You may drink a 16 oz. glass of juice rather than an 8 oz. glass for breakfast if you like.

Melon With Creme Sauce

One (1) Large Cantaloupe or Honeydew Melon

Cut melon in half. Put seeds and membranes in high-speed blender.

Cut each half of the melon into 6 or 7 wedges. With a sharp knife cull out the fruit from the rind. I slice the outer section of each wedge and cut into chunks and place in blender to fill up the blender jar. Cut the rest of each wedge into smaller pieces and put into 2 cereal bowls.

Blend seeds and fruit until smooth and creamy. Strain the sauce in a fine strainer over a large bowl, pressing out the juice. Discard the pulp. Pour sauce over the pieces in the 2 cereal bowls.

52

Basic Almond Milk

1 cup almonds soaked overnight
¾ cup pitted dates
1 tsp vanilla (optional)

Discard soak water and blend on high with 3 cups of distilled water. Strain through a fine sieve over a large bowl. Press out milk firmly with a serving spoon. (I save the pulp, dry it in the dehydrator, then put it in a container and freeze for future use.)

Pour milk back into blender and add the dates and vanilla. Blend and pour into 2 large glasses and enjoy! We like to use this recipe, or one using sesame seeds instead of almonds to accompany a bowl of sliced bananas.

Vanilla and Sesame Shake

¾ cup sesame seeds
3 cups distilled water
15 pitted dates (cut up and soaked if dry)
6 peeled bananas, cut in chunks
1 T. alcohol-free vanilla extract

Make sesame milk by blending sesame seeds with the 3 cups of water, strain through a fine strainer. Save pulp for future use. Pour half of the milk back into the blender, add half of the cut up dates, banana chunks, and vanilla. Blend well until smooth and creamy. This is one serving. Repeat with remaining ingredients for a second serving. Add crushed ice for a cooler drink.

Sesame Seed Nog

1 cup sesame seeds (soaked overnight)*
3 cups of distilled water
4 frozen bananas, divided, and cut into chunks
10 Medjool dates, divided, and cut up (soaked overnight if dry)
½ tsp nutmeg, divided
½ tsp ground cloves, divided
1 tsp alcohol-free vanilla extract. divided (optional)

Blend the sesame seeds with the water/date soak water and press the milk out in a fine sieve over a large bowl. (Discard pulp left in sieve or retain for future use in a dessert recipe. Spread out on a Teflex sheet and dry in dehydrator for several hours. Transfer to a closed container and put in freezer.)

Measure out half of the milk and return to the blender. Put half of the remaining ingredients in the blender and blend until smooth and creamy. This is one serving.

Place remaining ingredients into the blender and repeat the process. This is the second serving.

*Because I use a lot of sesame seeds, I soak three cups in a 1 ½ qt. bowl overnight, draining them in the morning and letting them dry. Then I have enough to last a while without having to soak for individual recipes.

Banana Leather

8 ripe bananas

Cut up bananas and place in blender. Run at high speed until all are liquefied. Pour onto Teflex sheets on dehydrator trays. Spread with a large spoon almost to the edges of the sheets to about 1/8 inch thick. Avoid having any holes in them. Dry at 105°F overnight or for about 9 hours. They should be pliable; do not allow them to get crispy. When ready the leathers will peel off easily from the Teflex sheets. Transfer them from the sheets to the plastic tray liners and turn them over to the smooth side. Using a sharp knife in one hand to hold the leather in place, tear into fourths or "quarters" with the other hand. Turn them over again to the rough side and roll each "quarter" into a tube. Place them on a large serving plate. Drizzle with Sweetened Strawberry Sauce.

Sweetened Strawberry Sauce

Use either a 1 lb. bag of defrosted unsweetened frozen strawberries or a 1 lb. box of rinsed, trimmed, and cut-up fresh strawberries. Add one third cup honey and blend in blender until smooth. Pour enough of the sauce to cover the banana leathers. Place in fridge overnight to soften. Eat with knife and fork.

Note: You may not need all the sauce—just save it for another time!

Whole Raw Fruit

Sometimes for breakfast we will just have fruit. For example, 4 oranges or 4 kiwis or cut up pineapple or papaya eaten in a bowl, etc. This is sufficient for Arlene, but Howard needs more. We have containers of raisins, figs, dates, almonds, cashews, pumpkin seeds, etc. on the table, which are readily available. Also on the table is a good supply of ripe bananas.

Banana – Papaya Pudding

½ large papaya, seeded and peeled, and cut into chunks
3 bananas peeled and cut into chunks
4 dried figs cut in pieces
½ cup water

Put papaya, bananas, figs and water into a blender and blend until smooth.

Lemon Pudding

2 avocados, cut in half lengthwise, pits removed and flesh
  scooped out
2 lemons, juiced
1 cup dates, pitted and soaked

Put everything in a blender and blend until smooth and creamy.

Banana Ice Cream

6-7 frozen bananas (peel bananas and freeze overnight in a
plastic bag; it helps to also put a large bowl and the
parts of the juicer that are used in the freezer overnight)
Using a Green Star or Champion juicer with the blank screen, process bananas into the bowl.

Ice cream can also be made in a food processor, but it will have to be made in several batches.

For toppings, make the Sweetened Strawberry Sauce found on page 55.

Or, for a "chocolate" flavor, try this:

1 c. maple syrup
½ c. raw carob powder
1/3 c. olive oil
1 T. alcohol-free vanilla

Blend all ingredients until smooth.
Try any other home-made fruit sauce for topping; or, just
plain maple syrup is good!

Since we are eating just 2 meals a day, the following recipes could come under the heading of Lunch, Dinner, or Supper!

Avocado Soup

2 tomatoes, diced
2 peeled garlic cloves, minced
2 ripe avocados (cut in half lengthwise, pit removed by
    stabbing with a small, sharp knife & meat scored
    with a knife to make small cubes)
1 stalk celery, thinly sliced
1 tsp. Celtic Sea Salt
1 carrot, grated
2 c. vegetarian soup stock (can be made by mixing 2 tsp.
    of dehydrated soup mix into 2 cups of water)
fresh or dried chives for garnish

Combine all ingredients in a blender and pulse to desired
consistency. This will leave some bits of vegetables in the
soup. Top with fresh or dried chives. Good with Crispy
Crackers.

Broccoli With Avocado Sauce

3½ c. broccoli, cut up into small pieces
1 avocado
2 T. fresh lemon juice
1 clove garlic
¼ c. 1st cold pressed extra-virgin olive oil
1 thin slice of jalapeño pepper or one or two sprinklings
½ tsp. sea salt   of cayenne powder
½ to 1 c. distilled water

Put cut up broccoli in large bowl. Blend the remaining ingredients in blender until creamy. Pour over broccoli and mix well. Marinate in refrigerator for 1 hour or longer. Top with parsley topping and serve with tomato slices.

Parsley Topping

½ c. onion, finely chopped
2 c. parsley, finely chopped
1/8 c. first cold-pressed extra-virgin olive oil
1 clove garlic, minced
1 T. fresh lemon juice
¼ tsp. Sea salt

Mix everything together and serve on top of the Broccoli with Avocado Sauce.

Colorful Tasty Veggie Mix

Use whatever vegetables you have on hand. We like a big variety of 1 cup diced: tomatoes, onion, celery, broccoli, portabella mushrooms, asparagus; 1 cup of corn cut off-the-cob, and 2 cups shredded carrots (or carrot pulp saved from carrot juicing).

Put all in a large glass bowl or casserole dish.

For Sauce, put in blender:

3 cut-up tomatoes	2 tsp. dried parsley
¾ c. olive oil	2 tsp. dried fennel
¾ c. distilled water	1 tsp. dried oregano
¾ c. lemon juice	2 tsp. minced ginger root
2 tsp. dried basil	2 tsp. Celtic Sea Salt

Blend well and pour over the vegetables. Mix thoroughly and dehydrate at 107° F for 4 or 5 hrs.

Confetti Corn Salad

Put all of the following in a large mixing bowl:

2 c. corn kernels cut from cob
1 c. chopped red bell pepper
1 large ripe tomato, diced
1 celery stalk, thinly sliced
½ c. thinly sliced green onions, or diced sweet red onion
¼ c. chopped cilantro

Dressing For Confetti Corn Salad

2 oz. Organic apple cider vinegar
2 oz. Bragg's or Nama Shoyu
2 oz. First cold-pressed extra-virgin olive oil
½ tsp. ground cumin

Put above ingredients in a jar and shake well. Pour dressing on top of salad and mix together.

Crispy Crackers

(This recipe is a little longer than usual, but will be worth it!)

2 c. almonds soaked 8 hrs. or overnight in distilled water and drained

1 c. sunflower seeds, soaked 8 hrs. or overnight in distilled water and drained

1 c. walnuts, soaked 4-6 hrs. in distilled water and drained

1 c. chopped onions

1 c. diced tomatoes

1 c. chopped celery

1 c. chopped red bell pepper

1 c. chopped carrot or carrot pulp from juicing carrots

1 T. cumin

3 T. ground flax seeds

½ T. Celtic Sea Salt

Put first eight ingredients in a food processor (may have to do several batches); or put in a heavy-duty juicer with the closed screen and remove the outlet adjusting knob. Have a large bowl to collect the dough. Add last three ingredients and mix well, adding enough distilled water to make a moist consistency. Spread out 1/4 inch thick on dehydrator shelves lined with Teflex sheets, and going up about 1 inch from the corners of the sheets. Score with dull knife or metal spatula to make 25 squares. Put in dehydrator at 105° F for 20 hrs, turning over midway. Check for doneness. If not dry, keep in dehydrator longer. If dry, remove tray and place another screencd tray (without the Teflex sheet) on top. Flip over and peel Teflex sheet from crackers. Put back in dehydrator. Let reverse side dry for 10 hrs. more, or until crispy. Store in glass jar.

Guacamole

2 ripe avocados, halved & pitted
¼ c. onion, diced
1 stalk celery, diced
1 garlic clove, minced
2 T. lemon juice
½ red pepper, diced
1 tsp. Celtic Sea Salt or Himalayan Crystal Salt
1 large tomato, diced

Scoop out meat from avocados & place in large bowl. Use potato masher to mash avocados to smooth consistency. Add rest of ingredients & thoroughly mix. Cover & chill in refrigerator. Serve in cabbage or romaine lettuce leaves, on crackers, or by itself.

"Fried" Mushrooms

2 large Portabella Mushrooms
½ T. minced ginger root
1 T. lemon juice
1 clove garlic
½ c. First cold-pressed extra-virgin olive oil
A little less than ¼ c. Bragg's or Nama Shoyu*

Clean mushrooms with a wet paper towel and dry. Remove stem from each mushroom and cut in pieces.

Blend remaining ingredients until smooth and pour in a large bowl. Add the stem pieces and the mushroom caps stem-side down for 30 minutes. Turn mushrooms over and marinate another 30 minutes. Place caps stem-side up on a Teflex-lined dehydrator sheet & pour some of the sauce inside the mushroom caps.

Dehydrate at 105° F for 2 hrs. or until soft.

*Nama Shoyu is a raw, unpasteurized Japanese soy sauce, but it contains wheat. For a non-wheat, unpasteurized product, choose Bragg's Liquid Aminos which is also unheated and unfermented, and is similar in taste and appearance to soy sauce.

Mushroom Burgers

2 large Portabella Mushrooms, cleaned and dried
1 avocado, washed & cut in half lengthwise, pit removed
Large slices of tomato and onion, lightly salted
2 dark green lettuce leaf halves
2 dinner plates

Slice the tops off the Portabellas, being careful not to cut too deeply so as to make a hole in the lower part. Turn the lower part upside down on a dinner plate. (This is the bottom part of the "bun." And the part that was cut off will be the top.) Spread the avocado on both inside parts of each mushroom. Put slice of tomato on top of the avocado on bottom portion of mushroom; slice of onion on top of the tomatoes; and top it off with a lettuce half. Put the top on and you're in for a real treat! This can be eaten in hand or, if it breaks up, use knife & fork.

NOTE: Usually there is a stem in the Portabella which must be removed. I cut off a thin slice of the outside of it and discard; then cut up the rest of it on the plate, along with some tomato and onion pieces and spread it with avocado. Yum!

65

Raw Spaghetti

For this I use a handy gadget called a "Spirooli." (www.buyspirooli.com).

Use the plate with the blade and small openings.
3 medium straight zucchini or yellow summer squash

Wash and peel zucchini or summer squash if not organic. Cut off ends. Fasten the fruit between the small circular opening and the prongs on the handle. Turn handle, pushing it forward, until it stops. Remove the end and long center from the machine. I use these cut up in salads. I like to cut the spaghetti into bite-size pieces, but you might like to leave it long.

Spaghetti Sauce

3 c. fresh tomatoes
1 c. cut up Portabella Mushrooms
2 garlic cloves
3¼ tsp. Italian Seasoning
¾ tsp. Celtic Sea Salt or Himalayan Crystal Salt

Put all ingredients in blender. Blend until desired consistency. You may want to leave it a bit chunky. Pour over Raw Spaghetti. Top with Rawmesan Cheese. Serve at room temperature.

Rawmesan Cheese

1 c. walnuts
1 c. nutritional yeast

Put above ingredients in food processor or blender & blend together. Add sea salt to taste.

Simple Paté

3 c. sunflower seeds, soaked overnight
1 clove garlic, minced
1/3 c. Bragg's or Nama Shoyu
2/3 c. fresh lemon juice

In a food processor or a heavy-duty juicer with the closed screen, process the sunflower seeds and garlic. Mix the lemon juice with the Bragg's or Nama Shoyu and pour into container with the processed sunflower seeds. Mix thoroughly with a large (serving) fork. Spread on large Romaine lettuce leaves, and top with slices of tomato and onion. Either fold over as a sandwich, or eat open-face.

Mock Tuna Paté

3 c. walnuts, soaked at least 3 hrs. and drained
3 c. carrot pulp (or shredded carrots)
1 T. lemon juice
1 c. celery, finely chopped
½ medium onion, finely chopped
1 or 2 cloves garlic, peeled and minced
½ c. cilantro, finely chopped
½ tsp. cumin
1 tsp. dried basil
1 tsp. sea salt

Process until smooth the walnuts & carrots in a juicer with a closed screen, or in a food processor (add a little water).

Add remaining ingredients and mix well. Serve in Romaine lettuce leaves.

This can also be made into crackers, spreading it on Teflex sheets and drying in dehydrator for 20 hrs., turning over midway.

Vegetable Plate With "Cheese" Dip

An array of assorted vegetables arranged attractively on a large plate, cut in sticks, circles, or left whole. Some suggestions:

> carrot sticks or baby carrots
> celery sticks, cut thin
> broccoli stalks, cut thin
> broccoli florets
> green onions
> radishes
> zucchini, or yellow squash, cut into rounds
> cucumber rounds or sticks
> red bell pepper sticks
> grape or cherry tomatoes, halved

"Cheese" Dip

> 1 c. walnuts or cashews, ground in blender
> ¼ c. fresh lemon juice
> 1/8 c. Nama Shoyu or Bragg's Liquid aminos
> 2 peeled garlic cloves
> ½ red bell pepper, seeded & roughly chopped

Remove ground nuts from the blender & put into a small bowl. Put remaining ingredients in blender in the above order, adding the ground nuts last. Blend until smooth and creamy. Put in small bowl & serve with Vegetable Plate. Refrigerating the dip for a couple of hours will thicken it.

Sometimes we will opt for a great big salad with lots of veggies in it and maybe half an apple or some raisins besides.

Here is our Favorite Sweet/Sour Dressing

Put in a 16 oz. Jar:

>½ c. olive oil
>slightly less than 1/3 c. organic apple cider
>>vinegar
>
>distilled water (about 2 oz.)
>1 clove garlic, minced
>½ tsp. Celtic Sea Salt
>honey to taste

Put lid on jar and shake vigorously until the honey is mixed in. Taste to see if sweet enough. Pour over vegetable salad and mix thoroughly. You may also want to add a favorite herb.

Here is another of our favorite dressings:

Green Dressing

¾ c. distilled water
¼ c. lemon juice
1/3 c. olive oil
1 garlic clove, halved

1 or 2 bananas
1 lg. handful fresh parsley
¾ tsp, sea salt

Put all ingredients in blender and blend until smooth. Pour

dressing over any vegetable salad. Yum!

Sour Cream Dressing

> 1 c. sesame seeds, soaked overnight & drained
> 1 T. fresh lemon juice
> 1 clove garlic, minced
> 1 tsp. Celtic Sea Salt
> 1-1½ c. distilled water

Blend all ingredients until smooth. Pour into bowl and garnish with chopped chives (fresh or dried). This dressing will thicken in the refrigerator. Can also be used as a dip.

Snack Food

> 3 c. sunflower seeds, soaked overnight and drained
> 1 c. almonds, soaked overnight and drained
> 1 large onion, diced
> 1 T. garlic powder
> 2 T. First cold-pressed extra-virgin olive oil
> 2-3 T. Nama Shoyu or Bragg's Liquid Aminos

Put the garlic powder, olive oil, and Nama Shoyu or Bragg's in a large bowl and mix together. Add the sunflower seeds, almonds and diced onion and marinate for 4 hrs. Spread on dehydrator trays lined with Teflex sheets and dehydrate at 100° F for 36 hrs. or until completely dry.

Our desserts are sweet and very satisfying.

DESSERTS

Date Bars

1 c. pecans
2 c. pitted dates
2 c. raisins
2 tsp. alcohol-free vanilla
2 c. dried unsweetened coconut (divided)

In a food processor or blender, grind pecans into a flour. Add dates, raisins and vanilla. Blend or process until it becomes dough-like. (In a blender you may have to add a bit of distilled water.) Remove from blender or food processor and put into a large mixing bowl. Work in 1/2 c. of the coconut with a large (serving) fork. Sprinkle 3/4 c. coconut in an 8" x 12" glass dish. Spread the date mixture on top of the coconut, and sprinkle the remaining 3/4 c. coconut on top. Cover and place in refrigerator. When cold cut into 48 - 1" x 2" bars.

Raw Carrot Cake

2 c. sesame seed or almond "flour" (made from the pulp
left over after making sesame seed or almond
milk. I save the pulp and dehydrate it until dry,
freeze in a container until I have enough for a
recipe, then grind the frozen pulp in a blender and
measure out 2 c.)

2 c. carrot pulp (from juicing carrots)

2 c. pitted dates, cut up (if dry, soak overnight. Save soak
water.) I use the large Medjool dates. It takes 12-13
to make 1 c.

1 c. chopped walnuts

2 tsp. alcohol-free vanilla

3 T. honey

½ tsp. Celtic Sea Salt

2 tsp. cinnamon

¼ tsp cloves

Enough distilled water (or soak water from the dates) to
make all ingredients stick together.

Put the 2 c. of cut-up dates in the blender with soak water
or enough distilled water to make a thin syrup.   Mix all
ingredients well in a large mixing bowl, using a large
(serving) fork. Flatten out dough in the bottom of the bowl,
divide in half with a spatula, and form a circular layer on a
large cake plate, using ½ of the dough. Freeze. Make
frosting.

Cover bottom layer of cake with frosting and put in freezer.

73

When frosting is hard, form the remaining dough on top of the frosting. Frost top and sides. Return to freezer.

Frosting For Carrot Cake

2 c. walnuts
1 tsp. alcohol-free vanilla
1 c. pitted dates
distilled water

Blend until smooth the walnuts and vanilla with enough water for the blender to work. Add the dates one at a time, using more water if necessary to get to right consistency.

Optional frosting

2 c. cashews
1 c. honey
1 T. Cinnamon

Blend cashews first until fine. Add the honey and cinnamon, and blend again until thick and creamy.

Coconut Frosting

1 ½ cashew pieces
½ C. coconut oil (or cocon. butter warmed to a liquid)
¼ C. maple syrup
2 tsp. alcohol-free vanilla
¼ tsp. sea salt
1/3 c. distilled water

Blend all ingredients until creamy.

Mock Marbled Cheesecake

3 c. cashews, soaked
¾ c. fresh lemon juice
¾ c. honey
¾ c. coconut oil (or coconut butter warmed to a
    liquid)
1 T. alcohol-free vanilla
¼ tsp. Celtic Sea Salt
distilled water, ½ -3/4 c.

Place cashews in the blender and grind fine. Add rest of ingredients and blend until smooth. Pour into a 9 inch spring-form pan. Drop the pan 1 - 2 inches from the table to remove air bubbles.

Blend 1 lb. fresh (rinsed and trimmed) or frozen strawberries with honey to taste. Scoop out several tablespoons and swirl into the cheesecake mixture. Reserve rest of strawberry sauce for topping individual pieces. Put pan in freezer until firm. Remove the sides of the spring form pan while frozen and defrost in refrigerator.

References

Baird, Lori and Julie Rodwell. *The Complete Book of Raw Food.* Long Island City: Healthy Living Books, Hatherleigh Press, 2004. www.healthylivingbooks.com

Boutenko, Victoria. *12 Steps to Raw Food.* Ashland, FL: Raw Family Publishing, 2001. www.RawFamily.com

Cohen, Alissa. *Living on Live Food.* Deerfield Beach, FL: Cohen Publishing Company, 2004.www.AlissaCohen.co

Letendre, Jalissa. *The Delights of Living Food.* Montreal: Jalinis Publishing, 2003. www.jalinis.com

Malkmus, Rhonda J. *Recipes for Life from God's Garden.* Shelby, NC: Hallelujah Acres Publishing, 1998. www.hacres.com

Nungesser, Charles and Stephen Malachi. *How We All Went Raw.* Mesa, AZ: In the Beginning Health Ministry, 2003.

Shannon, Nomi. *The Raw Gourmet.* Burnaby, BC, Can.: Alive Books, 1999.

Mail Order Resources

The Date People
P. O. Box 808
Niland, CA 92257
(760) 359-3211
datepeople.net
A husband and wife team
who grow over 50 varieties
of rare and exotic dates.

Jaffe Bros.
P. O. Box 498
Valley Center, CA 92082-0636
(877) 975-2333
OrganicFruitsandNuts.com
This is where I order my
unhulled sesame seeds,
Thompson Seedless
Raisins, Black Mission Figs,
and Solana Gold Apple
Cider Vinegar.

Sun Organic Farm
411 S. Las Posas Rd.
San Marcos, CA 02078
(888) 269-9888
www.Sunorganic.com

This is where I order my
large Medjool dates, also
Calamata olives.